What you
Chronic Obstructive
Pulmonary Disease (COPD)

By Kenneth Wright

In consultation with Dr Roger Matchett, the National Heart, Lung, and Blood Institute (NHLBI), the Global Initiative for COPD, and the Agency for Healthcare Research and Quality AHRQ, as well as our thanks to Dr. Peter Calverley, Dr. Thomas Petty and dr. Andrew Brown.

The publisher, Mediscript Communications Inc.acknowledges the financial support of the Government of Canada through the Book Publishing Industry Development Program (BPIDP) for our publishing activities.

ISBN # 978-1896616032
COPD, Lung problems, COPD patient education, preventing COPD, managing COPD.

Printed in Canada

IMPORTANT MESSAGE FROM THE PUBLISHER

A note of caution
This book provides generic information in harmony with the various medical authoritative bodies involved with Chronic Obstructive Pulmonary Disease (COPD). The information is basic and is intended to provide a general awareness of COPD and some coping suggestions when someone has COPD.

It must be emphasized that the prevention of COPD and the caring of COPD patients are wide ranging and depend on the health care practitioner's assessment of the situation. An accurate diagnosis with an assessment of the type and severity of the patient's condition by the health care practitioner is essential in the treatment of the patient.

Consequently, it must be absolutely made clear that this book is not a substitute for the health care practitioners advice and treatment to a patient or caregiver or family member of the patient. Any actions taken by the patient or cargiver or family member of the patient should be first checked out with the appropriate health care practitioner.

With this in mind the publisher and authors disclaim any responsibility for any adverse effects resulting directly or indirectly from suggestions, content, undetected errors or from misunderstandings on the part of the reader.

To order more copies of the book email mediscript30@yahoo.ca or telephone 1 800 773 5088 or fax 1 800 639 3186.

Table of Contents

ABOUT COPD

WHAT IS COPD?

You may have COPD if you have trouble breathing or you have a cough that will not go away. COPD is a condition that affects the lungs and airways, or bronchial tubes.

COPD stands for Chronic Obstructive Pulmonary Disease.

Chronic means it won't go away – you will have it the rest of your life.
Pulmonary means in your lungs.
Obstructive means partly blocked. The flow of air into and out of your lungs is limited.

COPD cannot be fully reversed. About 15 million people in the North America have COPD. It is the world's fourth leading cause of death; approximately 130,000 North Americans die each year from COPD – that is one death every 4 minutes. And an additional 12 million Americans and 1.4 million Canadians likely have the disease but don't know it.

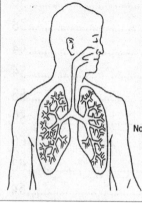

Normally, airways carry air to the lungs. These airways get smaller and smaller like branches of a tree. At the end of each tiny branch there are many small air sacs, like tiny balloons.

Normal lungs

In healthy people, each airway is clear and open. Each tiny air sac fills up with air. Then the air quickly goes out.

When you have COPD there are problems with this process, as follows:

1. The openings of the airways are smaller. Less air gets in because:
The walls of the airways get thick and swollen.
The airways are squeezed by small muscles around them.
The airways make mucus that you cough up.

2. The tiny air sacs cannot empty and your lungs feel very full.

The bottom line of all this is that the smallest airways, which are called the bronchioles, weaken and become less able to stretch. When you exhale, these very small airways may collapse before they empty out. Then even more air is trapped in the air sacs and, as you might expect, you have problems breathing.

It is worth emphasizing that the disease (airflow limitation) is usually both progressive and associated with an abnormal inflammatory response of the lungs to cigarette smoke or other noxious particles or gases.

Other breathing problems do exist, such as asthma, bronchitis and emphysema. Global Initiative for COPD, which is the authoritative medical body for the disease, clearly differentiates between these diseases and COPD.

Some symptoms of asthma may be similar to COPD, i.e. wheezing and difficulty breathing, but there are major differences in that with asthma the airflow limitation is reversible, the symptoms vary from day to day and you can have asthma even if you don't smoke. Also, the lungs may work normally between attacks of asthma and the person may be free of symptoms, which isn't the case with COPD.

Although chronic bronchitis and emphysema both have breathing problems as symptoms, the Global Initiative for COPD, in its definition of COPD does not use the terms chronic bronchitis and emphysema and excludes asthma.

CAUSES OF COPD - ARE YOU AT RISK?

Smoking

Smoking cigarettes is the most common risk factor for COPD, and causes 80 - 90% of all COPD. The earlier in life you start smoking and the more cigarettes you smoke each day, the more likely you are to develop COPD. So, the best way to slow the progress of COPD is to STOP SMOKING.

Pipes, cigars and other types of tobacco smoking are also causes of COPD.

Second hand smoke

If someone smokes in a family, this can contribute to the other members of the household developing COPD.

Indoor air pollution

The fumes from fuel used for cooking and heating in poorly ventilated dwellings can be a cause of COPD.

Outdoor air pollution

This factor can add to the lungs' total burden of inhaled particles and can be a contributing factor, although its specific role in causing COPD is not fully understood.

Occupational dusts and chemicals

These can be vapors, irritants and fumes. The exposure has to be sufficiently intense and prolonged.

Severe chest illnesses

If you had these when you were a child, they could possibly predispose you to developing COPD as an adult.

Over-sensitive airways

Having asthma or other respiratory illnesses can also be risk factors.

Heredity

In a small number of people, a rare genetic risk factor causes emphysema. These people lack alpha-1 antitrypsin, otherwise known as AAT deficiency. Their lungs are less able to protect against damage to the air sacs. COPD can run in families.

In summary, you absolutely know you are at risk if you smoke cigarettes or any tobacco product. There is a wide range of help available from physicians, pharmacists, health care professionals and counselors as well as products such as nicotine replacement therapy, drugs and other auxiliary products to help you quit.

If you are in the early stages of COPD, you have good reasons to be optimistic knowing that you can slow the progress of COPD, and live a longer and more enjoyable, unrestricted life simply by quitting smoking.

It is never too late to quit.

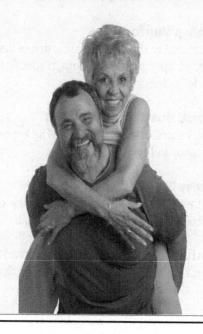

SYMPTOMS OF COPD

Notes

Coughing – "smokers cough"

Shortness of breath: usually gets worse during exercise, for example, when you walk upstairs

Excess sputum or phlegm

Feeling like you can't breathe

Can't take a deep breath

Wheezing

HOW IS COPD DIAGNOSED?

In order to determine whether you have COPD, your doctor will ask you about health problems, such as coughing, wheezing, amount of sputum, chest discomfort, severe chest illnesses, and shortness of breath. He or she will also ask about smoking and exposure to hazards in the environment and will give you a physical exam.

The physician's key clues or indicators for considering whether you have COPD are as follows:

History of tobacco smoking

Exposure to occupational dusts and chemicals

Smoke and fumes from home cooking and heating fuels

Shortness of breath that:
worsens over time (progressive)
Persistent (present every day)
Worsens with exercise
Worsens during respiratory infections

• Chronic cough
This cough may be present intermittently or every day. It can be present throughout the day but seldom only at night.

• Chronic sputum production
Any pattern of chronic sputum production may indicate COPD.

• Problems completing daily activities
Small tasks that use to be routine for you now become harder to complete.

• Acute bronchitis
Repeated episodes may be an indication of COPD.

Even though these indicators are clear, easy-to-recognize signs, adults can have COPD with no noticeable symptoms. Even with a few of these less severe symptoms, a person may blame a cough or a decline in fitness on aging or a smokers cough. Why not take this quick test?

Notes

	Yes	No
Are you a smoker or former smoker 40 years of age or older?	☐	☐
Do you have a cough with mucus that does not go away?	☐	☐
Do you get a lot of chest infections?	☐	☐
Do you become short of breath when doing a simple activity like climbing stairs?	☐	☐

If you answered "yes" to smoking or being a former smoker and one of any other question, you may be at risk for COPD. You should ask your physician for the breathing test called spirometry. This is a series of short tests that measure the amount of air coming in and out of your airways and lungs. These measurements help to identify whether COPD or another lung disease is causing your symptoms.

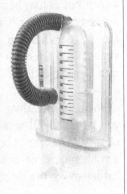

The spirometry test simply involves taking a measurement of the amount of air you can blow out of your lungs (a volume measurement) and how fast you can blow it out (a flow measurement). The spirometer reading can help your physician assess how well your lungs are working and determine the best course of treatment.

Notes

The spirometer records the results, and displays them on a graph for your physician to read.

You will be asked to take a deep breath, then blow out as hard and as fast as you can using a mouthpiece connected to the machine with tubing. The spirometer then measures the total amount of air exhaled, this is a volume measurement , called the forced vital capacity (FVC), and how much you exhaled in the first second, called the forced expiratory volume (FEV1), this is an air flow measurement.

When you have COPD there is typically a decrease in both the FEV1 and the ratio of FEV1/FEC. If your ratio of FEV1/FVC is less than 70%, then your COPD is classified as mild COPD.

In order to understand this a little easier, you can liken the diagnostic benefits of a spirometer to a blood pressure test. For example, blood pressure has 2 numbers (e.g. 120/80) measuring blood pressure during the heart beat cycle and indicates through the numbers whether or not there could be heart / blood circulatory problems.

In the same way, the FEV1/FVC measures the lung output providing a snapshot of lung health and efficiency. These spirometric results are expressed as a % predicted using appropriate normal values for the person's age, sex and height. For example you would expect very different results from a 24 year old athlete compared to a 6 year old child.

When the breathing ratios are low using a spirometer (when you have COPD), it means the lungs and airways have lost their elasticity and cannot bounce back like a healthy person – the way a rubber band or balloon does – and consequently it is much harder to get the air out.

COPD is classified as follows:

AT RISK Stage 0
Lung function is normal but chronic cough and sputum production are present. This is the ideal time to prevent COPD by stopping smoking.

MILD COPD Stage I
COPD is not too bad, with only mild airflow limitation. Even at this stage you may not be aware that your lung function is abnormal. However, you may cough a lot and feel a little out of breath if you work hard or walk rapidly.

MODERATE COPD Stage II
COPD is now getting bad. The limitation of airflow is worsening and there is definite shortness of breath on exertion. You may cough up more and you cough up mucus. You may take several weeks to recover from a chest infection. The symptoms can now have a serious impact on your quality of life.

SEVERE COPD Stage III
There is severe airflow limitation (you have trouble breathing day and night) or the presence of respiratory failure or clinical signs of right heart failure. Quality of life is seriously impaired and the exacerbations may be life-threatening.

Notes

CAN COPD BE PREVENTED?

YES COPD can be prevented in some cases simply by stopping smoking. Even in the early stages of COPD, stopping smoking will slow down its progression.

Of all the diseases that we experience, COPD is the easiest one for most people to prevent by getting rid of the causative factor – that is quitting smoking tobacco, be it cigarettes, pipes or cigars.

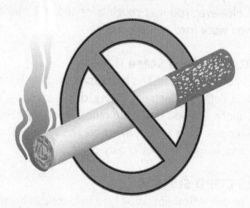

However, the truth is that once you have advanced COPD, physicians cannot cure COPD, but they can help to improve your symptoms and slow the damage to your lungs.

When you follow your physicians instructions:

- You will feel less short of breath.
- You will cough less.
- You will get stronger and get around better.
- You will be in a better mood.

WHAT I MUST DO
TO PREVENT COPD

Notes

_____

_____

_____

_____

_____

_____

_____

_____

_____

_____

_____

_____

_____

_____

IF YOU HAVE COPD

BREATHING TIPS

When you become short of breath, there are several methods you can use to help control your breathing. When you learn to control your breathing, you can get more air in and out of your lungs. The following methods can help:

Pursed-lip breathing

This method helps keep your air sacs and smallest airways open longer so that air is not trapped in your lungs. This helps stale air to get out of your lungs so more fresh air with oxygen can get in.

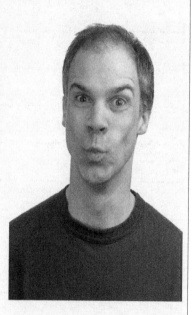

Follow these steps:

1. Breathe in slowly. This should be a normal breath (not a deep one). It is best to inhale through your nose, with your mouth closed. As you inhale, count "1, 2."

2. Pucker your lips in a whistling position. Now you have pursed lips.

3. Breathe out (exhale) slowly. Try to exhale twice as long as you inhaled. As you exhale, count "1, 2, 3, 4."

4. Relax.

5. Repeat these steps until you no longer feel short of breath. If you get dizzy, rest for a few breaths. Then begin again with Step 1.

Practice this breathing method several times each day so it becomes natural to you. Use pursed-lip breathing when you do things that make you short of breath, like climbing stairs, taking a bath, or doing housework. You also should use pursed-lip breathing for breathless spells.

Notes

Notes

Diaphragmatic (belly) breathing

The main muscle that we use to breathe is called the diaphragm. When you have COPD, air gets trapped in the air sacs in your lungs. The extra air makes your lungs push against your diaphragm. Diaphragmatic breathing helps make this muscle stronger, letting more fresh air into your lungs and getting the stale air out.

Follow these steps:

1. Place one hand on your belly, just below the ribs. Place the other hand on your chest.

2. Breathe in through your nose. As you inhale, let your belly and hand move out. Keep your upper chest relaxed. The hand on your chest should not move or move very little.

3. Purse your lips in a whistling position. Then breathe out slowly. Your hand and belly should move inward. Try to exhale twice as long as you inhaled.
4. Relax.

This method of breathing is harder to master than pursed-lip breathing. Practice each day as often as you think of it. At first, practice while you are lying down or sitting. Then begin to practice while you are walking. The more you do it, the easier it becomes. If you use diaphragmatic breathing daily while you talk, eat, bathe, and dress, your diaphragm will become stronger. A stronger diaphragm helps decrease your shortness of breath, strengthen your cough, and remove mucus.

Clearing mucus

Clearing mucus from your lungs will help keep the airways open and make it easier to breathe. This will help to prevent infections. There are a variety of methods and devices designed to help clear mucus. One method uses a special way to cough and is called controlled coughing. When you learn to control your cough, you can clear mucus more easily.

Follow these steps:

1. Sit in a chair with your feet flat on the floor. Hold a pillow against your diaphragm (upper belly).

2. Breathe in and breathe out through your nose slowly and deeply.

3. Repeat the above step 3 to 4 times.

4. Inhale again, bend forward, and push the pillow against your belly. Cough 2 or 3 times while pushing against your belly.

5. Relax.

6. Repeat as needed to clear your mucus.

Notes

Other methods and devices

Some people have very large amounts of mucus and cannot clear their lungs just by coughing. In this case, a method called postural drainage may help. Postural drainage uses gravity to help move the mucus. Your doctor also may tell you to use other methods, such as chest PT, which is short for chest physiotherapy. Devices that are available to help remove mucus include the Flutter device and the Acapella device.

Relaxation

When you become short of breath, it's very easy to panic. Shortness of breath causes fear and anxiety and eventually, panic can result. To help prevent this cycle, you can learn specific ways to relax. Try yoga, positive imagery (for example, picturing yourself in a pleasant place), and alternate tensing and relaxing of muscles. Diaphragmatic and pursed-lip breathing as previously explained, will also help you relax.

Tensing and relaxing your muscles

Follow these steps:

1. Sit upright in a chair, with your arms hanging loosely at your sides. Breathe deeply, slowly, and evenly.

2. Clench your fists while you continue to breathe.

3. Shrug your shoulders, and tighten your fists. Count "1, 2."

4. Let your shoulders fall down. Open your hands, and let your arms hang loosely. Count to 4.

5. Tighten your legs and feet. Count to 2.

6. Completely relax. Let all your muscles go loose. Count to 4.

7. Repeat as needed.

The way you sit or stand can sometimes make it easier to breathe. When you sit, lean slightly forward and rest your hands or forearms on your knees or over a table to support your upper body. When you stand, rest against a wall, leaning forward slightly. These positions help you avoid fatigue and shortness of breath.

SAVING ENERGY

You can learn ways to use less energy as you go about daily life. When you manage your energy better, it's easier to stay active. Adopting a slower, easier pace helps save your energy.

The 2 main ways to conserve energy are control of your breathing and planning your daily activities:

Breathing Control
As you learn to control your breathing, you'll feel more comfortable and be able to do more. Remember to use pursed-lip breathing and diaphragmatic breathing. When you carry out a physical task, do the hardest part of the work while you are breathing out.

Lifting: First, breathe in slowly. Then lift and place objects as you breathe out.

Pushing or pulling: First, breathe in slowly. Then push or pull objects as you breathe out. Repeat as needed.

Walking uphill or upstairs: Stop and breathe in slowly. Walk a few steps as you breathe out slowly. Keep your breathing even. Take the same number of steps each time you breathe out.

Daily Planning
You should wait about an hour after you eat before doing any physical activity. While your body uses oxygen and energy to digest food, you have less energy for physical activity.

Never plan a heavy day. Spread your chores over the week. Stop and rest often. Put a restful activity between activities that use a lot of energy. For example, you may get short of breath when you bathe and then dress right away. If so, bathe before breakfast, and dress after breakfast. If you live in a two-story home, plan ahead. Do what you need to do upstairs before you come downstairs.

Move everyday items close to the places where you use them. Gather items needed for a specific task to the same place. This way, you do not need to walk back and forth while doing the task. A small utility cart (with 3 shelves) can help you move things around as you do your tasks. A pair of tongs with long handles can help you reach for things. Remember to stop and rest often.

Notes

Think about using services in your community for help with meals, housework, and transportation.

Make each of the tasks you must perform easier. Don't stand when you can sit and don't hold your arms up when you can rest your arms. Here are some examples:

Cooking or ironing: Sit on a high stool, rather than standing.

Shaving or putting on makeup: Put a mirror on a table. Sit and rest your elbows.

Bathing: Use a bath seat. Wash your hair in the shower. A hand sprayer attached to your faucet or shower is helpful. Instead of towel drying, slip on a terry robe after bathing. Heat and humidity can also be a problem while bathing. Use your bathroom exhaust fan or leave the door open when you shower. Use a clear shower curtain if you feel closed in while showering.

Dressing: Wear loose-fitting clothes that do not restrict the movements of your chest or belly. Avoid socks or stockings with tight elastic bands that could restrict your blood flow. It's easier to put on shoes when you have slip-on shoes and a long shoehorn. Wear shoes with non-slip soles to avoid falls.

Notes

AVOIDING COPD TRIGGERS

It's important to take active steps to avoid activities and substances that can trigger flare-ups of COPD. The most common triggers are listed below:

Cigarette smoking: One of the most important steps you can take to control your disease is to STOP SMOKING. When you smoke, you breathe in poisonous substances such as carbon monoxide that stay in your lungs and airways and make your blood less able to carry oxygen. Smoke irritates your airways, which then may become inflamed and produce more mucus. Smoke also damages the cilia, tiny hairs that sweep the airways clear. When the cilia do not work, the airways become clogged with mucus and other matter. Clogged airways provide excellent conditions for infection to develop. Cigarette smoke also damages the air sacs in your lungs.

When you quit smoking – even though destroyed air sacs do not repair – your body starts to repair in other ways. When you quit, you slow the progress of COPD. The destroyed air sacs cannot repair themselves, but your body will start to repair in other ways. The cilia start to work again. When less harmful matter blocks your airways, air flow increases. More oxygen gets into your lungs, and more carbon dioxide is able to get out. Your lungs will work to clean themselves, so you may cough more for a while after you quit. Even if you have some lung damage, more oxygen will be carried to your body tissues. After you quit, you'll be better able to remove mucus from your airways and you'll have fewer infections and fewer periods when symptoms worsen.

In order to quit smoking, you need to do three things: prepare to quit, take action, and stay smoke free.

1. Prepare to quit.

Learn what is available to help you stop smoking. You may choose to quit "cold turkey," to use nicotine or non-nicotine medicines, to join quit-smoking classes, or all of these. Another name for quit-smoking is smoking cessation

Notes

Nicotine is a powerful drug that raises mood, reduces anxiety, and increases alertness. Nicotine causes changes in your brain that make your brain need nicotine. This is called addiction. When you try to quit smoking, the addiction causes you to have withdrawal symptoms.

The most common withdrawal symptoms are:

• lack of concentration

• irritability

• tiredness

• dizziness

• headaches

• craving for cigarettes

Today there are medicines that act as nicotine replacement when people are craving nicotine. Nicotine replacement comes as a gum, patch, nasal spray, inhaler, or lozenge. Also available is a non-nicotine medicine that works on the brain to produce some of the same effects as nicotine. Ask your doctor about these medicines.

Craving nicotine is not the only hard part of quitting. Most smokers have had daily smoking habits for a long time. To break the habit, you need to change the way you think about smoking. It's very helpful to develop a plan. Make a list of the times, places, and situations in which you usually smoke.

Here are 3 tips to break the habit:

1. Do something else during the times when you usually smoke.
Avoid tempting situations.
Stick with your effort.

2. Take action.

Set a quit date. Destroy all cigarettes the night before your quit date. Throw away all ashtrays, matches, and lighters. For several weeks, avoid the places where you usually smoked, if possible. Each time you get the urge to smoke, tell yourself that the urge will leave soon. Remind yourself why you want to quit. Try keeping your hands busy. Some people play with paper clips, doodle, handle a coin, or do crossword puzzles. If possible, get up and walk when you feel the urge to smoke. If you need to have something in your mouth, take sips of water, chew ice or sugarless gum, or eat fruit or a low-calorie snack.

3. Stay smoke free.

When you are tempted to smoke, ask for help from your family and friends. Employers, communities, and makers of nicotine and non-nicotine medicines may offer telephone support. There is no question that quitting is best for your health. Choose the plan that is best for you.

Infections: The flu and pneumonia are lung diseases that can be dangerous to you. You should get a flu shot every year in the autumn. The flu vaccine can prevent serious illness and death. Get the pneumonia vaccine as your doctor advises. If you had the pneumonia vaccine before age 65, and that was over 5 years ago, you should get the vaccine again.

To stay healthy, you need plenty of exercise, good food, and rest. Drink fluids to keep mucus thin. It is easier to clear thin mucus from your lungs and airways. Clear airways are less prone to infection. If you retain fluids or have heart failure, you must use caution in drinking fluids. Follow your doctor's advice about drinking fluids. And be sure to follow the rules of good hygiene:

Notes

•Wash your hands to avoid infections.

•Avoid crowded public places during the flu season.

•Avoid people who have the flu, a cold, or a sore throat.

•Keep your nebulizers and inhalers clean.

•Follow instructions for maintaining your oxygen equipment.

Call your doctor at the first sign of infection. The following are signs of infection:

•Your mucus changes in color, consistency, or amount.

•Your wheeze, cough, or shortness of breath gets worse.

•You get a fever or chills.

Air pollution: Outdoor and indoor air pollution in your lungs can trigger shortness of breath or lead to an infection. Avoid smoke, strong chemicals, and aerosol sprays. Use products that come as roll-ons, pump sprays, and liquids that are unscented. Avoid breathing in dust. Dust regularly with a damp cloth. If possible, have someone else do the heavy dusting and vacuuming.

Keep your furnace vents dust free. If you use an air cleaner, be sure you change the filter as the maker recommends. Keep your home free of molds.

During an air pollution or ozone alert, stay indoors, keep the windows closed if possible, and use a fan or air conditioner.

Avoid strenuous activity. Air pollution affects you more when you exercise or exert yourself. Breathing faster and deeper makes you inhale more air pollution. Ozone levels are highest in May through September, and are also are higher in the afternoon. If ozone levels create a problem for you, limit your outdoor activity to early morning and after sunset. If you react to pollen, stay indoors, keep windows closed, and use a fan or air conditioner on high-pollen days. Call your doctor if you develop breathing problems.

Weather: Cold air can be dry and irritating to the lungs. To warm the air you breathe, cover your nose and mouth with a mask or scarf, and breathe through your nose. If there's not a mask or scarf available, cup your hand, and keep it over your nose and mouth.

During the cold weather season, dry indoor air can be a problem. A continuous feed humidifier on your furnace can be helpful. Be sure you clean it as the maker recommends. It is best to keep indoor humidity at about 40 percent. Your doctor may advise you about other methods to keep indoor air moist.

During the summer months, heat and humidity may cause difficulty breathing. On hot, humid days, stay indoors and use an air conditioner. If your COPD includes asthma, you may need to be careful about allergies.

Second-hand smoke: Everyone should avoid second-hand smoke. Breathing second-hand smoke can change how the lungs and airways work. The airways may become more easily irritated. When people are exposed to second-hand smoke, their lungs may not work as well later in life. Do not allow smoking in your home. If anyone wants to smoke, ask him or her to smoke outside.

NUTRITION

Good nutrition means healthy eating. You need good nutrition to make your body stronger. You should eat a variety of foods every day. When you have COPD, preparing food and eating large meals may lead to shortness of breath. Here are some ways to help prevent shortness of breath:

Eat six small meals each day, instead of three large meals.

Chewing and digesting food uses up oxygen. When you eat a small meal, you use up less oxygen than when you eat a large meal. In addition, a large meal fills your stomach and a full stomach presses on your diaphragm. The diaphragm is the main muscle we use to breathe. When your stomach presses on your diaphragm, it is harder for you to breathe.

Eat foods that need little preparation.

Here are some of the foods that are both nutritious and easy to prepare:

• canned fruit and fruit juice

• fresh or dried fruit

• cereals, crackers

• cheese

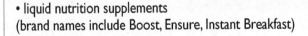

• eggs

• liquid nutrition supplements
(brand names include Boost, Ensure, Instant Breakfast)

• milk, yogurt, ice cream

- sandwiches

- tuna (salt-free)

If you are short of breath in the morning, plan a liquid breakfast. Eat slowly, and breathe evenly while you are chewing. Chew your foods well. If you feel the need, stop and relax. Take a few breaths. Then start again.

Avoid gas-forming foods. Some foods form gas that can cause pressure against your diaphragm. Avoid these foods:

- all beans (except green beans)

- broccoli

- brussels sprouts

- cabbage

- cauliflower

- cucumbers

- melons

- onions

- raw apples

- turnips

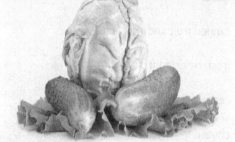

Ask your doctor for diet guidelines.

Some people may need to lose weight because extra weight can increase shortness of breath. Other people may need to gain weight. Your doctor will tell you the type of diet that is best for you or will refer you to a nutritionist. Other conditions you may have, such as diabetes or heart disease, will affect your diet guidelines.

If you feel the need for more help, you can ask your doctor to refer you to a nutritionist or dietitian. If you have a rapid gain or rapid loss in your weight, be sure to tell your doctor.

Notes

OXYGEN THERAPY

If there is not enough oxygen in your blood, your doctor will order oxygen for you. When there is too little oxygen in the blood, the heart starts to beat faster and harder to get more oxygen to the body's tissues. When the heart beats faster and harder over time, it may become damaged. Oxygen prevents heart damage and allows you to be more active.

When you do not have enough oxygen in your blood, you may have one or more of the following symptoms:

• shortness of breath

• tiredness

• irritability

• confusion

• headache

You may need oxygen but not have any symptoms. To decide if you need oxygen, the doctor will measure the amount of oxygen in your blood. A pulse oximeter measures oxygen through a clip on your finger or a sensor placed on your forehead. Another test, called a blood gas, uses a sample of your blood. Your doctor may also do further testing to learn what amounts of oxygen you need when resting, when active, and when asleep. Most health insurance plans require that you have these tests before they cover the cost of oxygen. Some insurance plans require a co-payment.

Oxygen Devices

Your doctor will prescribe the type of oxygen device, the flow rate, and how and when to use it. You should think of oxygen as a medicine. Use it as your doctor prescribes. You need to wear the oxygen as prescribed even when you feel fine. Talk to your doctor about changes in your oxygen prescription.

With any oxygen device, you can use 50 feet of tubing to move easily around your home. Be careful not to get caught or trip on the tubing. The following describes 3 types of oxygen devices:

Liquid: Liquid oxygen is the most portable type. This system is the easiest method for people with an active lifestyle. The device you carry weighs only about 7 pounds and allows you to move easily. You keep a base tank at home that must be refilled every 7 to 10 days. You fill the portable tank from the base tank as needed. How long the portable tank lasts depends on its size and the amount of oxygen you use. (The oxygen used is measured in liters per minute.) You must learn to plan ahead. You cannot let your portable tank become empty when you are away from the base tank.

Compressed gas: This type of oxygen is compressed into a cylinder and stored as a gas. The cylinders come in different sizes and must be replaced when almost empty. When you leave the house, there are smaller, portable cylinders of oxygen ("take-out" gas) to carry with you. You must plan ahead for how long the oxygen in your portable cylinder will last. Your home oxygen company will help you to calculate how much you need. In most cases, these cylinders cannot be refilled at home. They must be replaced. Be sure to store and safely secure all compressed oxygen cylinders.

Concentrator: This device stays in your home. It pulls oxygen from the air, concentrates it, and stores it. There is no need to have tanks refilled. Concentrators run on electricity and may increase your electric bill. Keep a compressed oxygen cylinder at home as a back-up in case of a power outage.

Traveling: Don't let your need for oxygen stop you from traveling. You can travel by air, car, bus, train, or boat when you plan ahead. Your doctor and home oxygen company can help you to arrange for travel. Before taking a plane trip, it's very important to talk to your doctor about extra oxygen for your flight. Special arrangements with the airline will be necessary. You also need to give advance notice for travel by bus, train, or cruise ship to arrange for oxygen with the carrier. You may need to get a prescription from your doctor. Request seating in a no-smoking area. For travel by car, do not allow smoking in the car.

Oxygen safety guidelines

Oxygen itself does not catch fire, but it supports fire. If anything near the oxygen source ignites, it will flame very quickly.

• Never smoke while you are wearing oxygen.

• Do not allow anyone to smoke around you. Put a "No Smoking" sign on your door.

• Do not use oxygen while cooking with an open flame. Appliances such as gas stoves, gas grills, and charcoal grills have an open flame. You can be very badly burned by an open flame that flares near oxygen. Talk to your doctor if you have an appliance with an open flame.

• Keep yourself and your oxygen equipment and tubing at least 5 feet away from any heat source that could ignite it. Some of these sources are hot pipes, candles, fireplaces, matches, stoves, and space heaters, even when not in use. Talk to your home oxygen supplier about a safe place and safe distance for your oxygen equipment in your home.

• Do not use appliances such as hair dryers or electric shavers that may create a spark while you are wearing oxygen.

• Be careful when you unplug any appliances while you are wearing oxygen.

- Do not use any oil-based creams or lotions, vapor rub, petroleum jelly, or hair dressings such as hair spray or gel when you are using oxygen.

- Do not use flammable products such as cleaning supplies or aerosol sprays while wearing oxygen.

- Do not store large amounts of paper, fabrics, or plastic near oxygen containers.

- Store oxygen containers upright in an open, well-ventilated area. Be sure the containers cannot tip over.

- In a car, secure the container in an upright position. Keep the windows cracked. Never store oxygen in the trunk or leave it unattended in the car – wear your oxygen.

- Be alert for kinks in your tubing.

- Avoid touching pipes and other metal parts on a liquid oxygen system – the frost may injure your skin.

- Install smoke detectors in your home. Check them regularly to be sure they are working.

- Store fire extinguishers where you can easily access them. Make sure they do not become outdated.

- Tell your local fire department that you have oxygen in your home.

These are general guidelines. It's also very important to know your particular oxygen system. Work with your oxygen supplier to learn about your equipment. Know its safety guidelines and how to use and care for it.

EXERCISE AND REHAB

You can benefit from exercise training at all stages of COPD. Exercise is important in order to build your endurance, strength, and flexibility. Some people try exercise and become short of breath, so they stop. They may think shortness of breath, fatigue, or muscle weakness makes exercise impossible. The truth is the less active you are, the weaker your muscles become. Your muscles then need more oxygen, and you become more short of breath. But you can work to get your body into better shape. Regular exercise can condition your muscles and make them more efficient. You then may feel less short of breath when you perform activities of daily living.

No matter how active or inactive a person is, exercise is important. You need to find an activity that is right for you. Pick an activity you enjoy, such as walking, dancing or stationary biking, then talk with your doctor about an exercise plan that may work for you. Ask how you should use your inhalers with exercise. Be sure to talk to your doctor before starting an exercise program.

When you exercise, you need to consider these important guidelines:

• Set up a regular program of exercise, and stay with it.

• Set goals that are realistic for you. This partly depends on how severe your COPD is. Start slowly. Some people may start only with 10 minutes of exercise once a day. Others may start with only 2 minutes a few times a day. Do what is right for you.

• Build up gradually. You can slowly increase your exercise time. Then you can slowly increase the intensity.

• Clear your lungs of mucus before each exercise period.

• Practice relaxation and deep breathing.

- Learn how you should use your inhalers before and during exercise.

- If you are prescribed oxygen with exercise, be sure to use it.

- Start your exercise period with a warm-up. Stretching and reaching are good ways to warm up. End the exercise period with cool-down activity. This means activity that is less intense or easier.

- Pay attention to what your body tells you. If you become very short of breath at any time, stop and relax. After a few minutes, resume your exercise.

- If your COPD flares up or worsens (exacerbates), your overall condition may decline. You may be unable to exercise at the same level. You will need to slowly work back to your prior condition and level of exercise. Follow your doctor's advice.

- If you become ill, reduce or stop exercise until your doctor says you may resume.

Many people start with a walking plan. To begin, you can start with a short walk each day. Go only as far as you can without shortness of breath. Keep your arms hanging loose and your shoulders relaxed. Some people find a walker helpful. It can support your arms or carry an oxygen device.

When you walk, breathe slowly, with your diaphragm. Use pursed-lip breathing: inhale 1-2, and then exhale 1-2-3-4. Keep the pace easy and even. Try to walk a little farther each day. Do not push too hard. When you become short of breath, always stop and rest.

Notes

MEDICINES

It's important to know that every medicine has 2 names – a generic name and a brand name. The generic name is the scientific name of the drug, while the brand name is the name that a specific company uses when it makes that drug. As an example, look at a common headache medicine. Many people use Ibubrofen for a headache. Ibubrofen is the generic name of the drug. The brand names include Motrin, Advil an Nuprin.

When your doctor prescribes a new medicine for you, you should review all of the medicines you take – both prescribed and over-the-counter – with your doctor. Every time you go to the doctor, take a list of all of your medicines with you, including inhalers. If your doctor changes your medicines and you start to feel side effects, call your doctor.

Medicines to treat COPD fall into several main groups:

Bronchodilators open airways to increase the flow of air. These medicines come as inhalers, nebulized liquids, and pills.

Short-Acting Bronchodilators
These drugs are short-acting bronchodilators that provide quick relief – they are fast-acting. They start to work in minutes, but last only 4 to 6 hours. These medicines are sometimes called "rescue medicines."

Keep one of these inhalers, if prescribed, with you at all times. Use it as prescribed when you have shortness of breath. If you need a fast-acting inhaler more than 12 times a day, call your doctor.

An increased use of rescue medicine may mean that your COPD is not well controlled. Possible side effects of fast-acting bronchodilators include faster heart beat, headache, and shaking (tremors). If you have side effects that bother you, talk to your doctor.

Long-Acting Inhaled Bronchodilators
Depending on the type, these last anywhere from 12 to 24 hours. Because these medicines help to keep your symptoms under control, they sometimes are called "controllers." They're also called "maintenance" bronchodilators. Usually these medicines are used on a regular basis (not "as needed"). They generally do not provide quick relief. Do not take them for an attack. They should not be used for immediate relief of breathing problems.

The 2 types of long-acting bronchodilators are beta-2 agonists and anticholinergics. Anticholinergic bronchodilators affect nerve impulses sent by the vagus nerve. When the vagus nerve is stimulated, the airways can narrow.

Oral Bronchodilators
Oral bronchodilators are taken by mouth. They are used to aid inhaled medicines. Oral bronchodilators work by relaxing the muscles around the airways.

Steroids
Steroids, which are another type of maintenance medicine, may reduce swelling and inflammation. These come in different forms, such as inhalers (both metered-dose inhalers and dry-powder inhalers), pills, and injections (shots).

Possible side effects of these medicines include hoarseness or a yeast infection in the mouth. There are several things you can do to avoid these side effects. Gargling with mouth wash or even water after taking these steroids helps to prevent side effects. If you use an MDI, attach a spacer to the inhaler.

Any steroid medicine may have side effects.

Possible side effects with short-term steroid use include:

• bigger appetite

• retaining fluids

• weight gain

• nausea or vomiting

• stomach upset or ulcers

• blood sugar changes

Possible side effects with long-term use include:

• high blood pressure

• thinning bones

• cataracts

• muscle weakness

• easier bruising

• slower wound healing

Oral steroids slow down the work of your adrenal glands. But when COPD symptoms suddenly get worse, oral or intravenous (IV) steroids are often needed. It's important to take steroids exactly as your doctor says.

Note: You can become seriously ill if you stop taking steroids suddenly. Do not stop taking any steroid medicines without talking to your doctor.

Notes

Combined inhaled medicines: Many inhaled medicines are available for COPD. Some people with COPD may need to take several of these medicines to manage their disease. To simplify taking these medicines, some have been combined into one inhaler. For example, some inhalers combine a maintenance (controller) inhaler and a rescue inhaler. Others combine 2 maintenance inhalers. Some combined inhalers include:

Expectorants and mucolytics: These are medicines that may help move secretions out of the lungs and airways. How well they work is not clear. For some people, drinking 6 to 8 glasses of water a day can have the same effect, and it costs less. Check with your doctor before trying this. If you retain fluids or have heart failure, you must be careful about drinking fluids.

Expectorants: These medicines increase fluid in your lungs and airways, and this helps secretions to liquefy and thin. They come as pills and liquids.

Mucolytics: These medicines break down mucus to make it easier to clear the lungs and airways.

Antibiotics: Antibiotics are used to treat infections caused by bacteria. Your doctor will choose medicine that is best to attack the kind of infection you have. It is very important to take all the medicine prescribed. If antibiotics are not taken as directed, the bacteria may become weakened, but not destroyed. This leads to antibiotic resistance. Always take antibiotics as your doctor says to destroy all the bacteria.

Notes

Always call your physician at the first sign of infection which could be:

• Your mucus changes in color, consistency, or amount.

• Your wheeze, cough, or shortness of breath gets worse.

• You get fever or chills.

Nebulizers: These are small machines that change liquid medicine into a fine mist. You then inhale the mist into your lungs. Many different nebulizers are on the market today. Directions for use are supplied by each company that makes these devices. To prevent infection, it is important to clean your device as the company recommends. Talk to your doctor about the best way for you to take inhaled medicines. Also check with your insurance company. Some insurance plans require a co-payment for nebulized medicines.

Inhalers

Inhaling is often the best way to take medicine for COPD. Inhaled medicines go directly to the airways and cause fewer side effects. There are several types of inhalers. Some common ones are the metered-dose inhaler (MDI), the Aerolizer inhaler, and the dry-powder inhalers (Diskus and Turbuhaler). The metered-dose inhaler has been available for years. The dry-powder inhaler and the Aerolizer are newer.

New devices come on the market all the time. It is very important to learn the correct way to use your inhaling device. For devices not in this booklet, be sure you get detailed instructions. Read the package insert, which may have printed instructions with diagrams. Also ask your health care team to watch how you use the inhaling device.

Metered-dose inhalers: There are 3 different methods for using metered-dose inhalers (MDIs):

• open-mouth method

• closed-mouth method

• spacer method

The spacer method is often preferred. A spacer deposits less medicine in your mouth and the back of your throat. With a spacer, you can inhale more medicine directly into your lungs, where you need it.

The next preferred method is the open-mouth method. When mastered, it leaves less medicine in your mouth and throat and more in your lungs.

It's important to become very familiar with the method you use. This will ensure that you get the most benefit from your medicine.

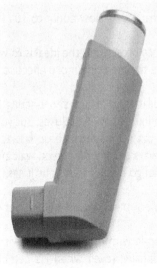

43

HOW TO USE INHALERS

Open-mouth method: Follow these steps:

1. Remove the cap. Hold the inhaler upright.

2. Check to be sure the mouth piece is free of any foreign object (such as a coin).

3. Shake the inhaler.

4. Tilt your head back slightly. Breathe out slowly.

5. Place the inhaler 1 to 2 inches in front of your open mouth (the width of 2 fingers).

6. Press down on the canister firmly as you start to breathe in slowly. (Press down until the medicine is released.)

7. Breathe in slowly for a count of 3 to 5 seconds.

8. Hold your breath for a slow count to 10 (10 seconds).

9. If more puffs are prescribed, the ideal is to wait between doses. This will make the medicine more effective.

• For bronchodilators that are short-acting beta agonists, it is best to wait 10 minutes between doses. But you may find it more practical to wait 3 to 5 minutes. These fast-acting inhalers begin to open your airways quickly. When you wait after your first dose, the next doses can go deeper into your lungs.

• For other inhalers, try to wait 1 minute between puffs.

10. Rinse and gargle with mouth wash or with water after using any steroid inhaler (even when it's combined with another medicine).

Note: If you carry your inhaler in a purse or pocket, make sure the cap stays secured. If the cap comes off, be sure to check the mouth piece for foreign objects (such as a coin) before you use the inhaler.

Notes

Closed-mouth method:
Note: This method is not preferred over the spacer or open-mouth methods. Less medicine reaches your airways with the closed-mouth method.

Follow these steps:

1. Remove the cap. Hold the inhaler upright.

2. Check to be sure the mouth piece is free of any foreign object (such as a coin).

3. Shake the inhaler.

4. Tilt your head back slightly. Breathe out slowly.

5. Place the inhaler in your mouth. Close your mouth.

6. Press down on the canister firmly as you start to breathe in slowly. (Press down until the medicine is released.)

7. Breathe in slowly for a count of 3 to 5 seconds.

8. Hold your breath for a slow count to 10 (10 seconds).

9. If more puffs are prescribed, the ideal is to wait between doses.

• For bronchodilators that are short-acting beta agonists, it is best to wait 10 minutes between doses. But you may find it more practical to wait 3 to 5 minutes. These fast-acting inhalers begin to open your airways quickly. When you wait after your first dose, the next doses can go deeper into your lungs.

Notes

• For other inhalers, try to wait 1 minute between puffs.

10. Rinse and gargle with mouth wash or with water after using any steroid inhaler (even when it's combined with another medicine).

Note: If you carry your inhaler in your purse or pocket, make sure the cap stays secured. If the cap comes off, be sure to check the mouth piece for foreign objects (such as a coin) before you use the inhaler.

Spacer method: Spacer devices offer several benefits. When you use a spacer, more medicine reaches your lungs, where you need it. Less medicine is deposited on your tongue and the back of your mouth. Side effects also are fewer and milder. For example, you will have less hoarseness and fewer mouth and throat reactions. If it's hard for you to compress the canister and inhale at the same time, your medicine dose may be more effective when you use a spacer.

There are several types of spacers available. It's important that you follow the instructions on the package insert for your particular spacer.

Follow these steps:

1. Remove the caps. Check to be sure the inhaler and spacer are free of any foreign object (such as a coin).

2. Attach the inhaler to the spacer.

3. Shake well.

4. Tilt your head back slightly. Sit upright, and breathe out normally.

5. Place the mouth piece into your mouth. Close your lips around it.

6. Press down on the canister firmly until the medicine is released. This will put 1 puff of the medicine into the spacer.

7. Breathe in slowly for a count of 3 to 5 seconds. Many spacers whistle if you inhale too fast.

8. Hold your breath for a slow count to 10 (10 seconds).

9. Remove the spacer from your mouth, and then breathe out slowly.

10. If more puffs are prescribed, the ideal is to wait between doses. This will make the medicine more effective.

• For bronchodilators that are short-acting beta agonists, it is best to wait 10 minutes between doses. But you may find it more practical to wait 3 to 5 minutes. These fast-acting inhalers begin to open your airways quickly. When you wait after your first dose, the next doses can go deeper into your lungs.

• For other inhalers, try to wait 1 minute between puffs.

11. Rinse and gargle with mouth wash or with water after using any steroid inhaler (even when it's combined with another medicine).

Note: If you carry your inhaler and spacer in your purse or pocket, make sure the caps stay secured. If the cap comes off, be sure that the inhaler and spacer are free of foreign objects (such as a coin) before use.

Doses left: You can use the math method below to find out how much medicine is left in your MDI.

Notes

Number of days: To find out the number of days that you can use a new MDI, follow the steps below:

Each inhaler is marked with the number of doses it contains. Find the number of doses marked on your inhaler. Example: 200 doses (or puffs)

Add up the number of puffs you use each day. Example: 2 puffs in the morning plus 2 puffs in the evening = 4 puffs per day

Take the number of doses (puffs) marked on your new inhaler. Divide it by the number of puffs you use each day. Example: 200 doses (puffs) divided by 4 puffs = 50 days of use

Take the number of days of use in your new inhaler. On your calendar, count that number of days ahead from the first day you will use the inhaler. Mark the date on your calendar that shows when the inhaler will be empty. Refill your inhaler prescription a day or two before the target empty date. Also, write the target empty date on the canister with an indelible marker.

Number of doses: To find out the number of doses left in your MDI, follow the steps below:

Count the number of puffs you have used from one inhaler for a certain number of days. Example: 4 puffs per day times 40 days =160 puffs used

Subtract the number of puffs used from the total doses (puffs) marked on the inhaler. Example: 200 doses (puffs) minus 160 puffs used = 40 puffs left

Divide the number of puffs left by the number of puffs you will use each day. Example: 40 puffs left divided by 4 puffs per day = 10 days of use left

The math method works only if you take a set number of puffs every day from your inhaler. If you use your inhaler "as needed," this method does not work.

Notes

There is a device on the market that attaches to your canister and counts the number of doses used.

CARE OF YOUR INHALER

Metered-dose inhalers: Rinse the mouth piece (plastic housing) and cap daily in warm running water. Wash the mouth piece and cap in mild soap and rinse in warm water at least 2 times a week, and more often if you have an infection. The mouth piece and cap must be dry before you use the inhaler again. While the cleaned inhaler is drying, you must use another inhaler.

Spacers: Clean your spacer well. Follow the instructions on the package insert for your specific spacer.

Dry-powder inhaler: The Diskus is a dry-powder inhaler. Follow these steps:

Hold the Diskus with one hand.

Place your thumb on the thumb grip. Then push it as far away from you as it will go. You will now see the mouth piece.

Slide the "trigger" away from you until you hear it click. Your dose is now ready to be inhaled.

Bring the Diskus opening up to your mouth. Be careful not to tilt the Diskus. It must stay in a level position until after you inhale the medicine.

Place the Diskus opening up to your mouth. Take in a slow, deep breath. As you breathe in, count to 5. This allows you to breathe all the medicine into your airways.

Hold your breath for up to 10 seconds. Move the Diskus away from your mouth.

Breathe out slowly.

Close the Diskus by sliding the thumb grip back over the mouth piece.

Rinse and gargle with diluted mouth wash, or just with water if you're not able to use mouth wash. This helps prevent hoarseness and an infection in your mouth from the inhaled steroids.

Never wash the Diskus after use. You may wipe it with a clean, damp cloth to remove any residue. The Diskus must always be kept dry.

Doses left: A counter on top of the Diskus shows how many doses are left. Each time you click the trigger, 1 dose is released, and the counter reduces by 1.

Many people use several inhalers at a time. You may wonder which inhaler you should use first. Keep in mind that bronchodilators work faster than inhaled steroids. Use bronchodilators first because these fast-acting inhalers open your airways quickly. Use the inhaled steroids last, so then they can go deeper into your lungs.

The general rules are:

• First, use your fastest-acting bronchodilator, for example, albuterol.

• Next, use any other bronchodilators prescribed for your regular use, for example, Atrovent.

• Last, use your steroid inhaler.

Gargling: It's very important that you rinse and gargle after you use inhaled steroids. Rinse and gargle with mouth wash or just water after using any steroid inhaler (even when it's combined with another medicine). This will prevent unwanted side effects that may occur with inhaled steroid use. One of these side effects is called oral thrush. If your mouth or tongue become sore or

Notes

reddened, call your doctor. You may need special medicine to treat this condition.

Follow-up visits

You will have regular doctor visits to see if your treatment plan is helping you. Your doctor will make sure you're doing all you can to prevent problems, including getting annual flu and pneumonia shots. How often you see your doctor for follow-up visits depends on your needs. Write down the treatment plan your doctor tells you to follow and remember to follow it at all times, even when you feel well.

When should you seek help?

If any of the following occur, get medical care:

• Your mucus changes in color, consistency, or amount.

• Your wheeze, cough, or shortness of breath gets worse, even after you take your medicine and it has had time to work.

• Your breathing gets difficult.

• You have trouble walking or talking.

Your COPD Treatment Plan

(Include all medicines: oral, inhaled, oxygen, over the counter.)

Medicine Name/Strength	Date Started	Purpose

Your COPD Treatment Plan

(Include all medicines: oral, inhaled, oxygen, over the counter.)

How to Take/ Time to Take	Other Info	Side Effects

Your COPD Treatment Plan

(Include all medicines: oral, inhaled, oxygen, over the counter.)

Medicine Name/Strength	Date Started	Purpose

Your COPD Treatment Plan

(Include all medicines: oral, inhaled, oxygen, over the counter.)

How to Take/ Time to Take	Other Info	Side Effects

Doctor Visits

• Write down questions and concerns to discuss with your doctor on your next visit.

• When your doctor prescribes a new medicine, ask if any other medicine should be stopped or changed.

• Take all of your medicines, including your inhalers, with you to each doctor visit.

Flu vaccine: _____   Pneumonia vaccine: _____

Special Instructions: _____

Nutrition Plan:

Exercise & Rehab Plan:

NOTES

NOTES

USEFUL WEBSITES

The Canadian Lung Association
www.lung.ca

The Global initiative for COPD
www.goldcopd.com

Sponsored patient information site
www.copdhelp.ca

Patient support website
www.copd-support1.com

Patient information from the UK
www.patient.co.uk

The US Lung Association
www.lungusa.org

Call 911
Right Away
if any of the following occur:

• You get confused.

• You have trouble staying awake.

• Your lips or fingernails are blue or gray.

Made in the USA
Middletown, DE
17 March 2023

26970126R00036